RickDixon Publishers
BD10 Bradford, West Yorkshire UK
First published in the UK

10 9 8 7 6 5 4 3 2 1

For written permission please write to RickDixon Publishers,
16 Summerbridge Drive, Bradford, West Yorkshire BD10 0ER, UK

Names have been changed to protect peoples identity and confidentiality.

Thomas P Benn other work

Whiskey House

About The Author

Thomas Benn has worked in supported living with people with learning difficulties, people with mental heath issues & worked with children ages 7 - 22 with autism.

As an experienced support worker with people with mental disorders has written this book on a subject dear to his hear. Thomas finds autism the most interesting and diverse condition there is. There is so much diversity that there is no end in learning about this subject. As you all learn from this book, Thomas continues to study the subject as it is of massive interest to the author.

Thomas only hopes that you please enjoy this book and that you learn and learn to understand autism.

Contents

Introduction

In the 1900s the word autism was taken from the Greek word autos meaning self. Autism is described by professionals as a complex pervasive developmental disorder. From my experience with working with people with autism, not one person is the same. I gained a mass interest in the subject due to it's massive diversity and individualism. To this day diagnosing autism is a challenge as some people only have minor signs and some have a trait that most other people have such as organizing or an intense interest or obsession with something. Autism affects many people in different ways.

Here's some history on autism:

- The first known reference to an autistic-like condition was in 1798 when it was used in relation to feral children.
- During the 1940s there was much debate as to the definition of autism.
- During the 1970s, Lorna Wing worked to define autism using the *triad of impairments.*
- During the 1990s research went into the causes of autism, several theories were published.
- The present day sees much more money going into research and development of treatments.

Autism is know among professionals as autism-spectrum disorder (ASD) as every person diagnosed with autism is placed on an autistic spectrum which helps to determine how the individual has been affected by autism. Is it minor or severe. The most common sign someone has autism is through their social behaviour. 90% of people with autism find it difficult to interact within a social situation. Some find it uncomfortable which can bring out certain behaviours, some can behave inappropriately as they do not understand what is appropriate in public as to being in private as at home.

Autism-spectrum disorder is not a bad or negative thing. It just takes time to understand the individual and learn what you can from them. Some people with autism can astound and amaze with the things they can do. I know I, for one are sometimes quite envious of some of their talents.

Causes Of Autism

Many different people have many different theories on the causes of autism. The truth is that there are many "possible" causes for autism. There have been millions of pounds/dollars spent on research each year but as of yet researchers and clinicians are still unable to establish a definitive cause.

Genetics

Some people believe it has to do with genetics, but this has not been proven. Some believe it is related to genetic abnormalities or that it is hereditary. There is some research that points towards genetic deletion, duplication or inversion as possible causes. Copy Number Variations (CNVs) are spontaneous alterations in the genetic maternal during cell division necessary for sexual reproduction, in 2009 this was a major focus of research. Researchers are still looking into a genetic cause for autism but as yet it is all coming back without solid proof.

Developmental

Other people believe that autism is caused during the developmental stages of a persons youth. Autism-spectrum disorder (ASD) tends to be diagnosed around the ages of 2-4 years. During this stage a child develops their cognitive, social, psychological and language skills. Parenting along with environmental, chemical and dietary factors can all affect development. Many people that have been diagnosed with autism have been missed diagnosed, as someone with autism can have traits that are similar to a child or mood swings like a teenager. The earlier the diagnosis the better, but to be more sure keep an eye out for the typical teenage/child like behaviour staying around into early adulthood.

Parenting

Some people still believe that poor parenting causes autism which is 100% not true, this has been proven. The theory linking autism with poor parenting was first published in 1943 by Leo Kanner. It's based on the premise that not showing a child love or affection increases self-adoration behaviours that can be associated with autism. It was believed by medical professionals and remained unchallenged until the 1960s! This has still to this day never been proven that this is a potential cause.

Vaccines

This is still a thing people believe today despite it being proven that vaccines cannot cause any form or amount of autism. The MMR triple vaccine (for Measles, Mumps and Rubella) was at one time believed to be linked to autism. Many parents to this very day still refuse to allow their children to be immunised, which is madness. Even though, the theory is now largely discredited. The MMR vaccine has been proven to have no relationship to the onset of autism.

Other Causes
- Mercury Theory – Higher levels of mercury in the blood
- Leaky Gut Syndrome – Gastrointestinal Disturbances that affect a childs development.

Other Untrue Causes People Believe
- Wild Boar Theory – The reduction of the body's intake of protein that helps brain function.
- Rain – The amount of rainfall affecting prenatal development.
- Lead – Lead poisoning during early child development.
- Paracetamol – This mainly replaced Aspirin in the USA in the 1990s. At the same time autism cases rose. This was pure coincidental.

In reality there is no clear explanation as to the cause of autism. Whether or not research is able to establish any substantial or definitive cause remains to be seen.

Autism fact: Males tend to be diagnosed with autism more than women. The population of people with autism stands at 60% male and 40% female.

The Diagnosis Of Autism

When diagnosing autism, there is no standard test or diagnosis procedure. Instead characteristic traits are used to identify someone with autism-spectrum disorder.

Here is a list of some examples of autistic traits:

- Little or no eye contact
- No fears or sense of danger
- Sustained play
- Over/under sensitivity
- Sameness
- Resistance of touch
- Language deficit
- Spinning/Tapping

Over the years, many types of autism have been described. It is now described as a spectrum that ranges from mild to severe. We refer to someone having an autistic spectrum disorder (ASD). Autism is very individual and so each person will be affected in different ways.

Asperger's Syndrome
First described in 1944 by Hans Asperger with regard to children in his practice who displayed:
- Lack of empathy
- Physical Clumsiness
- Non-verbal communication

The following behaviours are often associated with Asperger's Syndrome. However, they are seldom present in any one individual and vary in degree.

- ◆ Limited or inappropriate social interactions.
- ◆ Robot like or repetitive speech.
- ◆ Challenges with non verbal communication (gestures, facial expressions, etc.) coupled with average to above verbal skills.
- ◆ Tenancy to discuss self rather than others.
- ◆ Inability to understand social/emotional issues or non-literal phrases.
- ◆ Lack of eye contact or reciprocal conversation.
- ◆ Obsession with specific, often unusual, topics or subjects.
- ◆ One-sided conversations.
- ◆ Awkward moments and/or mannerisms.

It is still debated today due to it's similarity with high functioning autism. Someone with Asperger's syndrome will likely have good memories and usually have average or above intelligence, they will also have restricted interests which can be obsessive and also restricted behaviours. They have a huge love of routines.

Childhood Disintegrative Disorder
This is sometimes known as Heller's syndrome, first described in 1908. The child appears to develop normally until the age of two and then appears to regress in two or more of the following skills:

- Language
- Social function
- Communication
- Play
- Motor skills
- Bowel or bladder control

Once again someone with CDD can and will regress at various ages and rate, it is very individual. CDD is sometimes referred to as low functioning autism. Some medical professionals recognise it as being a separate condition.

Hyperlexia
A condition almost always in boys where autistic symptoms are accompanied by an excellent capacity for rote reading. By 2 years for age, these children have the ability to name letters and numbers, then by age 3 they may read printed words, exceeding even their ability to talk and by age 5 have a fascination with the printed word. Sometimes it's a talent I wish I had.

Some behaviours associated with Hyperlexia listed below. Remember to keep in mind that the severity, frequency and grouping of the following traits will differ with every individual.

- ◆ A precocious ability to read words far above what would be expected at a child's age.
- ◆ Child may appear gifted in some areas and extremely deficient in others.
- ◆ Significant difficulty in understanding verbal language.
- ◆ Difficulty in socializing and interacting appropriately with people.
- ◆ Abnormal and awkward social skills.
- ◆ Specific or unusual fears.
- ◆ Fixation with letters or numbers.
- ◆ Echolalia (repetition or echoing of a word or phrase just spoken by another person).
- ◆ Memorization of sentence structures without understanding the meaning.
- ◆ An intense need to keep routines, difficulty with transitions, realistic

behaviour.

Savant Syndrome
This is a rare form of autism that effects less than 10% of autistic individuals. The person has extraordinary skills unlike that of any other person. These are usually related to memory, mathematics, art or music. For examples of people with Savant Syndrome look up Daniel Tammet, he is a mathematical savant who can do some of the worlds most challenging equations in his head in mere seconds. Also look up Kim Peek, the 'real Rain Man'. The cause is unknown although there are many unproven theories.

Associated traits are:

◆ Some people with Savant Syndrome can appear 'slow' mentally.
◆ Some individuals can have an unrealistic, superpower like memories (eg. Look at a map for mere seconds and remember every detail for years)
◆ Superhuman ability to do any form of mathematical equation, from calender dates to extreme equations.

Rett Syndrome
A neuro-developmental disorder first described by Andreas Rett in 1966. The clinical features include:
• A deceleration of the rate of head growth and small hands and feet.
• Stereotypic, repetitive hand movements such as mouthing or wringing are also noted.
• 80% of females have seizures
• They typically have no verbal skills

Rett syndrome is known as high functioning autism.

Attention Deficit Hyperactive Disorder (ADHD)
This is probably one most people have heard of. This is a very common form of autism. Let's try something a little different here.

Have you ever had trouble concentrating, found it hard to sit still, interrupted others during a conversation or acted impulsively without thinking things through? Can you recall times when you daydreamed or had difficulty focusing on the task at hand?

Most of us can picture acting this way from time to time. But for some people these and other exasperating behaviours are uncontrollable, persistently affecting their day to day existence and interfering with their ability to form lasting friendships or succeed in school. With care and attention a parent/carer can easily learn to give someone with ADHD a happy normal life. You know them, now start thinking.

The Triad Of Impairments

The triad of impairments is a widely used tool to describe, diagnose and understand autism-spectrum disorder. It was first described by Wing and Gould in 1979. It shows how people with autism have trouble in three different areas.

- Social Communication
- Social Interaction
- Social Imagination

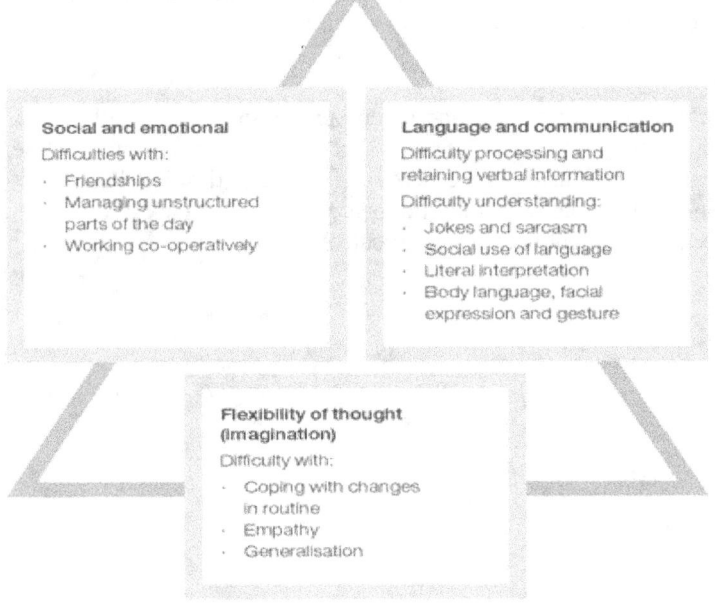

Social and emotional

Difficulties with:
- Friendships
- Managing unstructured parts of the day
- Working co-operatively

Language and communication

Difficulty processing and retaining verbal information

Difficulty understanding:
- Jokes and sarcasm
- Social use of language
- Literal interpretation
- Body language, facial expression and gesture

Flexibility of thought (imagination)

Difficulty with:
- Coping with changes in routine
- Empathy
- Generalisation

Social Communication

People with autism have difficulty using and understanding verbal and non-verbal language, such as gestures, facial expressions and tone of voice, as well as jokes and sarcasm. Some people with autism might not speak or have fairly limited speech. They may understand what people say to them but prefer to use alternative forms of communication, such as sign language. Some people with autism find it too uncomfortable in conversation that they might change the subject completely mid sentence to a subject they know a lot about or feel comfortable with, this is normally one of their obsessions. Here are some conversational tips when talking to an autistic person, keep in mind they may not all work as each person is very individual.

- Talk in third person, it helps stop confusion
- Do not say NO, use maybe or later
- Try not to use nicknames as this can cause confusion
- Use short simple words to communicate to help with understanding
- Body language is very important. Place your feet shoulder width apart and keep arms down by your side relaxed.

Social Interaction

People with autism have difficulty recognising and understanding people's feelings and managing their own feelings. They may, for example, stand too close to another person, prefer to be alone, behave inappropriately and may not seek comfort from another person. This can make it hard for them to make friends.

Social Imagination

People with autism have difficulty understanding and predicting other people's intentions and behaviour and imagining situations that are outside their own routine. This can mean they carry out a narrow, repetitive range of activities. But keeping mind that a lack of social imagination should not be confused with lack of imagination, many people with autism are very creative.

Key Effects of autism

Sensory processing and sensory sensitivities
People with autism often perceive or process sensory stimulation or information differently to non-autistic people. Hyper-and/or Hypo-sensitivities are common. An autistic person often have extreme senses for example, a bright light may only make a non-autistic person screw their eyes up for a second, an autistic person may see that light ten times more bright. This also works with sound, pain and smell. It has actually been proven that someone who is hyper-sensitive to smell can actually fell pain, if someone wears a certain aftershave or perfume near that person, it can physically hurt them. This can also work the opposite way too, like not smelling a very strong smell.

Sensory Sensitivities
Hypersensitivities
- e.g. Light, noise, smell etc.
- Can be extremely diverse

Hyposensitivities
- e.g. Pain
- May be oblivious to an injury

Sequencing of information
People with autism often struggle to understand the order of events during the day for example. Some people have talked about every day being like a blank piece of paper. Often help with understanding the order in which things are done or the days programme is very helpful e.g. a pictorial or written timetable.

Predictability & Reliability
People with autism often find the world they live in an unpredictable and confusing place. This also applies to the actions and reactions or others. Sudden movements and sudden noises can startle them even if it is a continuous sound e.g. cuckoo clock that goes off every hour will still startle them every hour even though they have lived with that happening for years. Establishing and maintaining routines is important to helping establish a sense of reliability and control. We need to consider how we act and react, the more consistent the better.

Ritualistic Behaviours and Obsessions
Certain things are more important to people with autism. Something non-autistic people could find 'silly' is very serious to someone with autism, for example an autistic person might love bus times tables and must collect them and/or memorise them, if a new one come out they must get it as fast as they can or they can become

very uncomfortable and feel a loss of control. Finding some activity that is repetitive and absorbing can help block out unwanted stimuli. It can also help exert some control on the world around them, sometimes we call these safety behaviours. Trying to stop these behaviours might cause great distress even though they might be obstructive and prevent a person from engaging in other positive activities. Rather than stop, try to distract towards a favoured positive activity. Always reward and reinforce positive energy by being descriptive about what is good that the person has done. The frequency and intensity may relate to the persons level of anxiety, the more anxious the person is, the more likely they are to get 'stuck' in an obsession or ritualistic behaviour.

Communication
Developing a person centred individualised communication strategy is important. Most people with autism find verbal communication accompanied by visual communication more effective e.g. using pictures, signs or symbols to communicate along with spoken language. Creating a communication profile could be very important to help with communication between yourself and someone with autism. This will help make the autistic person be understood better and also help you communicate with the individual in a way they feel more comfortable with.

- Communication charts – recording how a person communicates, listening, observing, recording.
- Communication strategies – having clear individual plans in place for each person used by all who support them.
- Person centred support – find out how the individual likes and needs your support.

Understanding the social world, relationships and social norms
As we've seen from the triad, this is a key area of difficulty. People with autism will need support in learning to understand the social world. They may also need support in learning skills and understanding social boundaries. It is equally important that we accept that the people who need our support with managing their autism in every day to day life are unique individuals and not to expect them to understand the world and relationships in the same way that we do. Non-autistic people should adapt their approach in order to meet their needs like providing person centred support.

Person Centred Approach
A person centred approach means to deliver support in a way which is based on and suited to the individual's needs and choices. For example, when coming in to contact with or supporting an autistic person in social interaction we should consider
- The time and place for interaction – it needs to focus on the person's ability to cope in a given situation.
- Understanding the context of a situation is vital for the person with autism but is often over looked.

When and Where

People with autism don't like busy crowded places. This is usually due to the person's ability to process sensory information. Busy high streets for example are full of sensory stimulation such as lots of movement, colours and noises. This can sometimes overwhelm the person, cause anxiety, panic and result in behavioural changes.

Challenging Behaviour

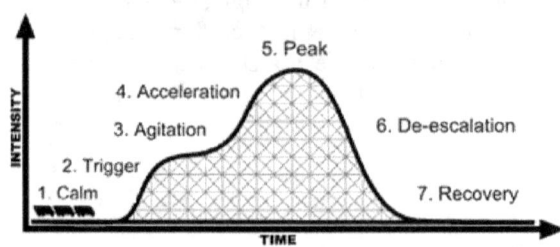

Above is a well used diagram known as the Challenging Behaviour Cycle which shows what happens when a person (even you and me) gets agitated or upset. Here's a brief description on what you see above.

1. Calm – That is a person at their usual, natural state.
2. Trigger – Is the thing that has upset us or caused us distress.
3. Agitation – This is us getting agitated.
4. Acceleration – This is us getting more and more distressed until we reach the Peak stage. Remember the more agitated someone gets, the less likely they are going to understand what is being said to them.
5. Peak – This is the moment when we will show challenging behaviours. We may lash out physically, shout or even throw things.
6. De-escalation – This is the moment when we begin to calm down. We are leaving the distressed state and making our way back to Calm.
7. Recovery – And this is when you have fully finished being upset and are generally back to your normal Calm state. This is a good time to talk about what got the person upset, then you can learn to remove the trigger and avoid the whole situation.

All individuals can behave in a challenging way, even you and me. But people with Autism-spectrum Disorder can seem more challenging than the average person due to lack of understanding of their condition. Look up the disorder your in need of information on and take notes, but remember, you know the individual better than any professional or doctor so you have a huge advantage. Here is a list of challenging behaviours that people with Autism tend to display more than us.

◆ Refuse or ignore requests.
◆ Behave in socially inappropriate ways, such as taking their clothes off in public.
◆ Become aggressive.
◆ Engage in self-stimulatory behaviour such as rocking or hand-flicking.
◆ Hurt themselves or other – for example, by head banging or biting.

Now, when experiencing these types of behaviours keep in mind that this is because the individual is agitated in some way. They tend not to behave in these ways because it takes their fancy. Here is a list of reasons someone with autism may act in this way, keep these in mind when trying to de-escalate the situation.

- Having trouble understanding what's happening around them – for example, what other people are saying or communicating through facial expressions and body language.
- Not having effective ways of communicating their own wants and needs, which leads to frustration.
- Feeling very anxious.
- Feeling uncomfortable with their surroundings, is the place too noisy, busy or bright?
- Having their routine effected.

Routines
People with Autism often like predictable environments and can get very upset if their familiar routines are broken. For example, the person might be upset if you change the route you usually take home from a regular visited place.

Transitions
People with ASD might not understand that it's time to move from one activity to another. Or with some people, they just might not want to.

Sensory Sensitivities
If the individual has sensory sensitivities they may like feeling or touching particular surfaces or materials. They may get upset if thy are unable to.

Sensory Overload
An individual might get upset if too much is happening around them, if a particular noise is overwhelming or it's too bright for them.

Unrealistic expectations
Any person with Autism can get frustrated if they're expected to do something they do not have the skills for, such as getting dressed by themselves.

Tiredness
People with autism-spectrum disorder have problems with sleep, and poor sleep can cause very difficult daytime behaviours.

Discomfort
This could include things like the feeling of clothes against skin, a prickly label, wet pants, a bump or pain. Check with your doctor if you suspect there could be a medical reason for the challenging behaviour.

Identifying what has caused the behaviour (Trigger)
If you notice an individual with autism is becoming agitated, try think about what made them upset. Was it something in the environment? something someone said to them? Has their routine been messed with in some way? Whatever the cause try think about how you could do things differently next time. Try removing the Trigger before it has a chance to escalate into challenging behaviours. This makes life easier for you and for the individual with autism. Try think about making some changes.

Making Changes
If you know something in the home or out and about will trigger challenging behaviours for an individual then try to change them. For example, if an individual does not like crowded place, do not go into town. Here are a list of things to think about.

- Organise predictable routines, perhaps using picture timetables.
- Prepare the individual for changing routines. For example, by giving the individual a five minute warning (using a clock is good) before stopping for breaks in routine. Using pictures is a good way to help the individual understand more clearly.
- Set up gradual introductions to environments that might be over stimulating. For example, start with short visits during which the individual gets something they like, or go when it's less busy.
- Communicate clearly with the person. Make sure the individual is paying attention when you tell them what's going to happen. Use only one request or instruction at a time. Use simple language (no slang) the individual understands. Pictures are particularly useful.
- Teach the individual how to ask for things they want or need (if they don't already).
- Plan for situations you know might be difficult. For example, don't do new things when the person is tired, or let them take a favourite item or theirs.
- Calmly ignore the persons protest (never ignore the person) but when they do something good, give them plenty of praise.

Other Considerations

Transfer of Knowledge

People with autism-spectrum disorder often rely on visual learning to understand information, we all use this process to some degree. Consistency and routine form a key part of how information is transferred. Inconsistency can lead to confusion and mixed results (he does it for Rick but not for me). A concise care plan can help.

Rigid Thinking

This is where a person can get locked into certain beliefs or ideas. Think of a skill like holding a pen, if we can do this, our brain will allow the concept to be expanded on into other areas such as drawing or painting. A person with autism often need help to expand on their already pre-existing skills.

The person or Behaviour

When helping or supporting someone with ritualistic behaviours, our focus should be on the person rather than what they are doing. If you were talking with your friends would you focus on the way they're dressed or what they are telling you? Always keep positive and focus on the positive things they are doing or saying. To someone with autism this is similar to a reward, they then try and use the behaviour that they were praised for over behaviours ignored. Gentle teaching can sometimes be used to support people with ritualistic behaviours.

Gentle Teaching – Key Principles

- Ignore/interrupt the behaviour not the person. This focuses attention on the person not what they are doing.
- Redirect the person to another activity such as getting a drink or a snack.
- Reward the person using social, descriptive praise such as "well done for pouring the drink well".

The most important things to be aware of while communicating with someone who has autism are these three things. These are very noticeable and important to someone with autism.

Communication is made up of: Body Language 60% Tone of Voice 35% words 5%

Eye Contact

This one is very individual as most people with autism do not like any form of eye contact but in some cases this is pleasant. There are many different theories on eye contact and it's importance in communication. Remember, how you use this depends on the person, and if you're family, a friend or a carer then no one knows the person like you do. The impact of eye contact can change depending on the situation. Does someone not looking at you make you feel like they are listening to you or ignoring you? But generally speaking, people with autism do not like prolonged eye contact.

Body Language
When in a general conversation, body language makes up over half of the message we receive. Imagine someone having a normal life conversation with you but they are facing away from you. Some body language is subconscious and beyond our control. While talking to someone with autism then it is best to keep your body as neutral as possible. For example:

- Feet shoulder width apart.
- Shoulders relaxed, not tensed up.
- Hands loose, placing just your thumb into your pants pocket is a good position.
- Feet facing the person you are communicating with, this shows you are paying attention to them.
- Never have your hand clenched or arms folded. This shows you are uncomfortable talking to the individual.

Tone of Voice
There are several components that make up the way we use speech, this could involve words, tone, volume etc. Some people believe that tone of voice makes up 35% of our communication.

Do
- Speak in you normal voice – not too quiet or loud
- Keep it simple, be clear, direct and reassuring.

Don't
- Try to speak too much or use complex sentences or questions
- Shout

Wording
The English language is full of multiple words with a similar meaning. How many words can you think of for having a cigarette or having a drink? We often assume that people understand our shared meaning. For people with autism it is important to be consistent in the language we use.

What to say and how to say it
Helpful:
- I can see you are upset
- How can I help?
- Let's go
- What's wrong?

- It'll be O.K.
- Would you like to...?
- Every thing's alright
- I understand
- Please...

Not helpful:

- Stop that!
- Don't....!
- Why....!
- You're being stupid!
- You're letting yourself down!
- Behave yourself!
- Stop making a fuss

Space
No, not our universe but personal space. How much personal space do most people need? Most average people only need and arms length, sometimes with someone with autism this can stretch to two arms lengths. If someone is angry or unset you might want to consider that this person may require more space than normal. Personal space should only change based on relationship status if the individual enjoys cuddles or closeness. But think about this, if you are angry, annoyed or just upset, do you want someone to come over to you and cuddle you? In normal circumstances it is hard for a person with autism to concentrate on everyday things as it is but being in their personal space is even more distracting. Imagine your sat in an arms chair reading when someone comes over and sits on the arm for a long period of time.

Living With Autism-Spectrum Disorder

Jennifer

When I was diagnosed with Asperger's Syndrome in 2006, I was shocked and paranoid. This made me do massive amounts of research and this helped me to understand certain things that had confused me throughout my life.

When I told my friends and family I had some strange comments like is it a disease, why didn't you tell me before. As for being a disease, no it's not, it's part of me and who I am. Would it have made a difference knowing about it, to me yes and it has already helped me to understand so much, but really I'm still the same person.

I now understand why I didn't understand certain things that seemed simple to others but that is just how I am wired but to the 'normal world' people with autism are viewed as outsiders. I once spoke to an autism specialist who said that he believes that autism is the next step in evolution. That made me feel really good because that would be so nice if that was true.

Jennifer

Benjamin

Hi I'm Ben. When I was diagnosed with autism I just shrugged it off and just another name the doctors have given to another problem and didn't take it seriously. I now understand why I feel weird in certain situations.

When I go to the pub to hang around with people I know I find it hard to instigate conversation. I find it easier if they talk to me and I can just reply 'yes' to what they're saying. Even though I've known these friends for years I still need 2 or 3 pints to be able to feel comfortable to approach them and start talking to them.

I always hang out at the same places because that's normal to me. If someone suggests we go somewhere else I have a mini panic within myself and would rather stay in the same place by myself than go somewhere strange to me with people I know.

I remember when I was 15 or so and I went shopping with my mother. I was thinking in my head that I needed some new jeans. Without saying anything to my mother, she suggested I get some new jeans, for some reason I became annoyed and told her 'I don't need any new jeans, there's fuck all wrong with these ones (the ones I had on)' I felt annoyed all day for some reason unknown to me. I made me more agitated because in my head I was thinking 'you wanted some new jeans so why didn't you just let her buy you some'. That is something that always puzzled me. I don't know if it was because she got in there first before I asked or what. I have trouble with things like that a lot of the time. I still hope that one day I will manage to control my awkwardness but I haven't got any closer as yet.

Ben

The Goth

I was giving a talk last year to assorted support workers when one of them asked me who, then, given my isolation in youth, I would turn to for someone to talk to and share my feelings with. Why would I want to share my feelings with anybody?

After four years of working in classrooms with autistic children, this person had not grasped what it means for someone to lack the drives necessary for instinctive socialisation — a thing I'm tempted to call a lack of socialism — but still went with assumptions about what autists think based on people in general. This is even more marked in people I know personally: as soon as the situation includes them they stop making allowances for me.

I call empathotypical people interactive tables; they display somewhat more complex behaviour, but they are objects in my world, a distinct group, but not special. They fail to stand out; this is in contrast to empathotypical behaviour, which gives people a special place in empathotypical thoughts and feelings — I don't know if I'm making any sense; I feel like I'm describing red to the congenitally blind.

I suspect that I use the same part of my brain to recognise all types of table, in contrast to the table-recognition skills of some tables (people), which are centred in a special area of the tabletop.

I lack instinctive socialism, but not a desire for social contact — I have been dogged by loneliness, driving people away through progressively more desperate attempts to attract attention. I lack instinctive empathy — at least for people — a lover of the finest craftsmanship, I don't own a Chippendale, but if I did, I wonder how the care I would lavish on it would differ. It would be less rewarding, more one-way, but would my affections underlying the care be the same?

I wonder if communication is a third thing, or just a consequence of socialisation and empathy. I don't lack ability with words, but I lack the impetus to learn in just the situations where I have most to learn.

I choose to concentrate my efforts in people; greater pros outweighing greater cons, but I recognise other autists who shy away from the problem of interacting, discouraged by the enormous effort which produces so little progress. It is a worthwhile and rewarding trek.

the Goth

Jane

ACCEPTANCE is the most important word in the entire vocabulary of the autism and neurotypical dialogue.

I am a female on the spectrum. I've always known it ever since I first heard the word autism. Sadly I have met no professional people who believe that I know what I am talking about. I have not been issued an official diagnosis. It makes me angry beyond words. They have no ACCEPTANCE. They think their piece of educational paper means they know more about my life than my 54 years of living it.

I am a very lonely person. I do have a husband but he is all the family I have. My natural family has never had any interest in being in my life. I was shuffled through the foster care system when I was growing up. That was a nightmare. None of those families had any idea who I was as a person. Even now as an adult I face rejection often. There is no ACCEPTANCE. I am expected to be normal. I can't because I'm not.

I love my autism. I have friends on Facebook who are mostly all on the spectrum. They don't turn their backs on me. We all recognize that we have what others might think of as weirdness. We also have trust. Autistic people are the only ones I trust. They put my mind at peace. They don't criticize or bully. They just want to be involved in whatever it is that holds their interest. We don't play superiority games. We are equals. Even if we can't relate to each other's interests, we don't knock anyone for having those interests. We have ACCEPTANCE of each other. Actually, I think this makes us infinitely more interesting.

I make an analogy of autistic people to geodes. Geodes are plain looking rocks until you open them up. Then you realize that they have spectacular natural treasures inside. No two are exactly alike but they are all beautiful beyond description.
The thing I want people to know about autism is that we are human. News media talks about us as if we are from another planet. Nope. We all have to share this one. In order to do that peacefully they have to learn ACCEPTANCE of us. Talk TO us not about us. Even more important, LISTEN.

Jane

Acknowledgements

After years of wanting to write this book but have been so confused on how to word things and make it easy to understand. I decided to keep it short and sweet and hope this helps at least one person understand themselves or the person they know. Autism is a good thing to live with as long as you understand the person with the diagnosis.

If you live with autism then just know never feel like an outcast, be proud, you can do anything anybody else can do.

Anyway to my thanks

I would like to thank everybody I've ever worked with with autism, you are amazing, all of you. I must give credit to Sheerwood Training for their training and knowledge you've passed onto me. Thanks to everyone who read this book and taking time to understand other peoples issues and needs and wanting to make life easier for them and yourself. Finally, I would like to thank the people who gave personal statements in the 'living with autism' chapter, it must hard to let others read what you feel.
Thank you.

www.ingramcontent.com/pod-product-compliance
Lightning Source LLC
Chambersburg PA
CBHW072253200526
45168CB00015B/1722